ALL YOU WANTE
Kriya

CW00985158

Ravindra Kumar, Ph.D.
(Swami Atmananda)

New Dawn

NEW DAWN
a division of Sterling Publishers (P) Ltd.
A-59, Okhla Industrial Area, Phase-II, New Delhi-110020
Tel : 6313023, 6320118, 6916209, 6916165
E-mail : ghai@nde.vsnl.net.in
www.sterlingpublishers.com

All You Wanted to Know About - Kriya Yoga
©2000, Sterling Publishers Private Limited
ISBN 81 207 2326 0
Reprint 2001

Published by Sterling Publishers Pvt. Ltd., New Delhi-110016
Lasertypeset by Vikas Compographics, New Delhi-110029.
Printed at VMR, New Delhi.

Contents

Preface

Kriya yoga is the most advanced technique amongst all disciplines of yoga. One can enter into it after about two years of *hatha yog* which purifies the body and calms the mind, which are the pre-requisites for kriya yoga. It is a combination of nearly 20 practices. Since it does not require the control of mind; which follows eventually automatically; it suits all kinds of practitioners -householders or recluse. It is a very effective method of experiencing Kundalini directly.

The basic text, with variations of course, has been dealt with by several writers, all of whom deserve thanks from us, especially Swami Satyanand Saraswati. However, the methods presented in this small book are a result of my personal experiences with Kundalini over the years. Having taught mathematics for more than 30 years in eight countries, I resigned as a professor in 1994, and dedicated myself fully to developing these practices at 'The Academy of Kundalini Yoga and Quantum Soul'. Thanks are due to Jytte Kumar Larsen for computing facilities and related help.

Swami Atmanand (Ravindra Kumar, Ph. D.)
Founder and President
Academy of Kundalini Yoga and Quantum Soul
58-61, Vashisht Park, Pankha Road,
New Delhi-110046.
Tel: 504 7091, 503 4143, 504 1368, 513 7567.

Introduction

Most of the ways for awakening the Kundalini require strict discipline, austerity, and dos and donts which are not so easy for an average person to observe. For these reasons the *yogis* thought and designed the kriya yoga practices which are free from most restrictions, but, nevertheless, are extremely effective. Kriya yoga awakens the chakras, purifies the nadis, and finally raises the dormant energy in a slow and safe manner. Abrupt

7

awakening can create situations at times which may be difficult to handle.

Mind is thought, to be an obstacle in the way of spirituality. But this is not so. Mind is the only vehicle which eventually brings higher consciousness on transcendence. Negative emotions like greed, lust, anger, attachment, ego, etc., should not be used against the mind for its condemnation. If energy is suppressed, it will explode in another way. What is required is the conversion of negative thinking into positive thinking. This is gradually achieved through kriya yoga practices. In a physical balance, the pan of negativity is lower than that of positivity, due to the gravity of negative thoughts. But the practices of kriya yoga slowly brings the other pan lower down.

The properties of any single *guna* (virtue) is not exalted: tamas, rajas or sattva as one of the *guna* dominates the other two. Even the most sattvic person shows signs of tamasic and rajasic activities at times. Even so, the most tamasic person shows signs of rajasic and sattvic properties at times. But the importance lies with the dominating virtue, of course. Gradual practise brings the transformation of the mind from inert, to scattered, to vacillating, to one-pointed, to a controlled one.

For ages, these teachings have been a secret, but they were not clearly defined. They were passed on from the teacher to the disciple. The methods are so powerful, that, if the person is not prepared to handle the aggravated situation, it can misfire and the person may have to go into an asylum. That is why a practice of *asanas*, *mudras* and *pranayam* is necessary for some time before commencing the advanced techniques. Kriya means practise or action, hence it is the yog of practise.

Hatha yoga practise is very essential in this regard and is recommended for a period of nearly two years to prepare a practitioner for advanced kriya yoga practices. It controls the vital energy *pran* which interacts with the mind; consequently, the mind is controlled with the control of *pran*. One achieves a tranquil and calm mind, even in the midst of disturbing circumstances, because of chemical secretions in the body. It is a permanent achievement, unlike a temporary one through LSD, etc.

Through kriya yoga one achieves the state of simultaneous awareness of worldly senses and objects on one hand, and inner tranquillity on the other. There is predominance of alpha waves in the brain which is responsible for stopping the movement of the mind. The aim of tantra is to expand the mind and liberate the energy.

The underlying principle of kriya yoga can be understood in two steps: generate the nectar and reverse its flow. Practices like *khechari mudra* are meant to stimulate the *bindu* and thus create nectar. The nectar, on being created normally, goes down to *manipur* and is burnt off. Practices like *vipareet karni* (opposite doing) are meant to reverse the flow of the nectar, so that, it is not wasted and is directed to higher centres for consumption in the body, which can arrest ageing and produce rejuvenation, This principle of reversal of flow is highlighted in the famous book *Hatha Yog Pradipika* and other tantric texts. The mind reaches the state of *shoonyata* (void or nothingness) and begins to act like a witness to everything happening around.

Left-Hand Path of Kundalini Tantra

Tantra is composed of *tanoti* (expansion) and *tranyanti* (liberation), meaning thereby, the science of expansion of mind and liberation of energy. Tantra endeavours at raising Kundalini by uniting the two opposites — Shiv and Shakti, through yogic practices. Shiv or *purush* is the masculine counterpart representing consciousness, and Shakti or *prakriti* is the feminine counterpart representing energy. These two

14

opposites are encountered in all spheres of existence; for example, man and woman in physical life, mind and pran in spiritual life, ida and pingla in hatha yoga, time and space in cosmos or on mental level, etc. The word Tantra — Hindu, Jain or Buddhist — came into existence some two thousand years ago. There are two main branches of tantra. They are, right-hand path or *dakshin marg* and the left-hand path or *vam marg*.

Right-hand path observes a high degree of purity in conduct and action, and makes use of the meditational and spiritual practices.

Left-hand path lays stress on the sex drive and believes that the sexual interaction between man and woman, representations of Shiv and Shakti in human life can raise the Kundalini. The fusion of the opposite forces results in an explosion and manifestation of the matter. The yogi is not interested in either procreation or pleasure but in *samadhi*. He/she generates an experience and sublimates it, opening thereby the gates to higher consciousness. This is the trick. Sexual life is combined with yogic practices to explode the energy. It is in the midst of the climax, as the attention is diverted from sensual pleasure to the thoughts of the Absolute, that the third-eye opens, without any notice or preparation. One gets a glimpse of the higher experience, of the reality, a taste of enlightenment.

The same elements which are responsible for the fall of a man, such as desires and passions, are transformed and used for liberation in the "left-hand path." Moralists and teachers of religion have always denounced sexual life, but it continues to exist. One may give it up, but it continues to remain in the mind, since it is perhaps the most powerful urge. Whether one lives a sexual life or as a celibate, in either case he/she can be spiritual or non-spiritual.

One endeavours at the extension of the period of sexual interaction through the use of hatha yoga practices, such as, siddhasana, vajrasana, vajroli/sahajoli mudra, tribandh (three locks) and pranayam, so that the semen is retained for a long time and ejaculation is delayed. More the extension of the period, greater the chances of enlightenment. While the experience is held, the retention of breath (*kumbhak*) directs the energy

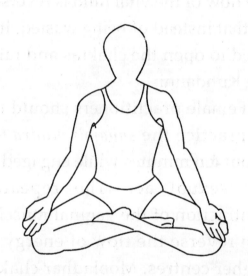

Siddhasana

to higher centres which pressurises them to open up. The direction of the flow of the vital fluid is reversed so that instead of being wasted, it is used to open the chakras and raise the Kundalini.

Female practitioners should try to practice the *sahajoli mudra* for about ten minutes while engaged in the sexual act. The repeated contraction of the vaginal muscles can reverse the flow of energy to higher centres. Mooladhar chakra (root centre) may be awakened and tantric orgasm may be experienced. She may transcend ordinary consciousness any time and may see

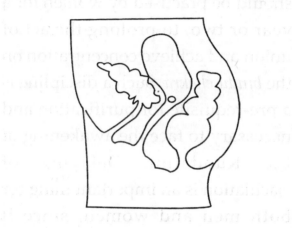

Points of concentration for females
Sahajoli Mudra (Clitoris, lower vaginal
muscles and urethra)

the light. Siddha-yoni-asana, vajrasana, tribandh, sahajoli mudra and other hatha yoga postures should be practised by women for a year or two, to prolong the act of union and achieve concentration on the *bindu chakra*. Such a discipline is a pre-requisite for purification and necessary to face the awakening of the Kundalini. Delaying of ejaculation is an important thing for both men and women, since it increases the frequency of the act, maintains the body temperature, and there is no feeling of depression. With sustained practise, enlightenment can be achieved. It is the fastest and easiest method, since people are used to the act, although some risks are involved, as discussed earlier.

Both man and woman should co-operate with each other with the prime goal in mind. The woman is respected as a goddess (*devi*) and not as the object of pleasure. This path is for serious minded householder practitioners who have practised the 'right-hand path' well and have achieved control on their passions; otherwise it can lead to their downfall.

Right-Hand Path of Kundalini Tantra

The Right Hand Path or *dakshin marg* does not involve sexual enactment. It had been the most widely followed method prior to the removal of barriers on sexual life. Now of course in the modern society, sexual drive is well recognized and *left-hand-path* is known to give fastest results, though proper care needs to be taken as risks are involved in it. Yet the age-old *right-hand-path* has its own importance because of its purity and risk-free methods of *kriya yog*.

The *divine energy* flashes consciously on its descent into the practitioner from the plane of pure consciousness (*Shiv*). It is called *shakti-pat* and is a sort of signal to the yogi that he is on the right path of evolution. It can be considered as an initiation after which the Kundalini does not descend back to the lower chakras, which it may otherwise do and the progress may be slow, since the Kundalini may pause at lower chakras.

Shakti-pat gives an intuitive consciousness to the yogi and he becomes aware of the rapid mental transformations. It is not a matter of right, but it takes place spontaneously when the practitioner has purified himself or herself through various yogic practices.

The biological organism is spiritually fortified and it resounds with the vibrations of the *mantras*. One can integrate oneself purposefully. One has partial omniscience of most of the events taking place in the universe.

Nadis and *chakras* play an important role in the awakening of the Kundalini and they have been discussed at length in a separate booklet of this kind. We will now introduce the *right-hand-path* of kriya yog.

Simultaneous Activation of all the Chakras

Kriya yoga is the most powerful method in the modern age and it is suitable for all kinds of people regardless of their lifestyles, habits or beliefs. It has been evolved by the tantric rishis for an easy adaptation by all since it does not involve any do's and do-not's. Following the yogic exercises are useful for the simultaneous activation of all the chakras and a preparation for the more advanced techniques of kriya yoga. These exercises can bring a transcendental state which is indescribable in words.

Exercise 1 : Meditation on Chakras
Sit comfortably in *siddhasana* or *siddha-yoni-asana* with eyes closed

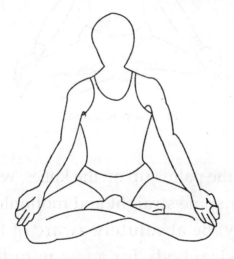

Siddhasana

29

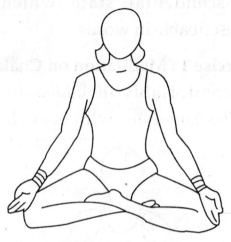

Siddha yoni asana

and the palms up on the knees, with
your spine straight and motionless
body. Be absolutely aware of the
physical body for a few minutes.
Shift your awareness to the spinal

column and then to the ajna chakra. Discover pulsation in ajna and become absolutely aware of it. Synchronize it with *Om-Om-Om-Om* which you should recite 20 times. Now remain in *ashwini mudra* (contracting and relaxing the anus) for about four minutes. Ajna centre will be automatically felt after few practises.

Now bring your awareness to mooladhar chakra and discover a pulsation there while counting 20 times. Open the eyes and gaze at the tip of the nose (*nasikagra mudra*) for about three minutes. Slowly you will be aware of both ajna and mooladhar. Bring awareness to swadhishthan chakra and discover a pulsation while counting 20 times. Practise now *vajroli/sahajoli mudra* (drawing up and releasing the genitals) for about four minutes.

Bring awareness to navel region, and to a psychic breath from mooladhar to navel, and from throat to navel. The two breaths should coincide at navel at the point of complete inhalation. Retaining the breath brings awareness to a central point in the navel region.

Release the breath and repeat the process for about four minutes.

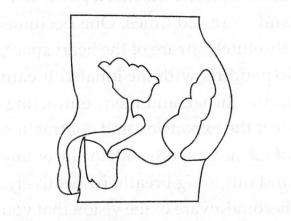

Points of concentration for males
Vajroli Mudra (Penis)

Bring your attention to the manipur chakra, find a pulse there and count 20 times. Move your awareness to the anahat chakra, find a pulse there and count 20 times. One becomes absolutely aware of the heart space, expanding with the inhaled breath in the throat, and then contracting. Feel the expansion and contraction of the heart space with the incoming and outgoing breath, respectively. Become aware of the vision that you might see in the heart space. Practice for two to three minutes. Now bring awareness to the throat pit and then to vishuddhi chakra, find a pulsation there and count 20 times.

Move consciousness in sushumna from mooladhar to swadhishthan, to manipur, to anahat ,to vishuddhi, to ajna, touching each chakra with an imaginary flower; and reverse the process from ajna to mooladhar similarly. Repeat the process five times and then chant *Om* for about a minute.

Exercise 2 : Fourth Order Pranayam

Sit in a comfortable and erect position, breathe deeper and deeper and fix your attention on the rhythmic flow of the breath, for a couple of minutes. Chant O while inhaling and M while exhaling thus synchronizing the mantra *Om* with the breath mentally. Pay attention to ajna and feel that you are inhaling with O and that the breath is piercing all the chakras, from mooladhar to swadhishthan, to manipur, to ajna, to vishuddhi, to ajna, to sahasrar. In the same way while exhaling with M feel that all the chakras are pierced back in the reverse order. Repeat the process a couple of times. Then bring attention to ajna and concentrate on O while inhaling through eyebrow centre, and on M while exhaling through it. Thus synchronize your awareness with *Om* for as long as you can.

Exercise 3 : Unmani Mudra

The literal meaning of *unmani* is 'no mind', that is, thoughtlessness; the state to which this exercise brings the practitioner. Sit in a comfortable position with body straight and eyes open. Concentrate on the *bindu* and breathe deeply. Feel that you are inhaling through bindu. While exhaling, shift your awareness from the bindu, to ajna, to vishuddhi, to anahat, to manipur, to swadhishthan, to mooladhar. Eyes should be closed as you exhale. Open the eyes and repeat the process 10 to 15 times. The eyelids will close spon-taneously. It is mainly a mental process.

Exercise 4 : Conduction of the Seed Mantra

The ascending psychic passage (*arohan*) begins from the mooladhar chakra to the swadhishthan area and then to the manipur area, following the curve of the belly. It then ascends to the anahat area, to vishuddhi area, to bindu, in a straight line path. Alternatively, one can carry awareness from the vishuddhi area to lalana chakra in the palate, to the tip of the nose, to the eyebrow centre, to sahasrar, following the curve of the skull and finally to the bindu. The descending passage (*awarohan*) goes down from the bindu, to ajna chakra, to vishuddhi, to anahat, to the manipur, to the swadhishthan and then to the mooladhar. Seed mantras at each centre from the mooladhar to the bindu are:

mooladhar ..... *lam*

swadhishthan ..... *vam*

manipur ..... *ram*

anahat ..... *yam*

vishuddhi ..... *ham*

ajna ..... *om*

bindu ..... *om*

Sit in siddhasana with your eyes closed and body straight. Bring attention to the mooladhar, chant *lam* once, and feel the pulsation. Let the attention jump to the swadhishthan area, chant *vam* once, and feel the pulsation. Travel this way to bindu. Return in the same way through each centre to mooladhar. From each centre the awareness should jump to the next. Normally ten rounds will be a good practise. One can devote more time at each centre, say for one to five minutes, if one likes to do that, with the chanting of corresponding mantras and feeling the vibrations.

The Yogic Sleep

Awareness of all the chakras can be very effectively developed through this method in the following steps:

- Lie down comfortably on a cushion in the death-pose (*shavasana*) — face and palms facing upwards, body straight and eyes closed. Make sure that the body will remain motionless throughout the exercise.

- Become aware of the space in front of the closed eyes, feel that the space has surrounded the whole body, and that you are fully immersed in it. Feel that the body has become as light as a feather, and that it is sinking into space. Practise this way for a couple of minutes.

- Bring awareness to the navel region and feel that you are inhaling and exhaling through the navel rhythmically, without altering the natural form of breathing.

- Resolve your spiritual aspiration through the feelings of the heart, repeating it a couple of times.

Feel that you are looking at your body from a distance - toes, legs, knees, thighs, pelvic region, abdomen, chest, arms, hands, fingers, shoulders, neck, mouth, face, nose, ears, eyes, eyebrows, infact, the body as a whole. Repeat the process, starting from the toes again and visualizing every part, for a couple of minutes.

Discover and develop awareness of each chakra. Begin with the mooladhar situated between the anus and genitals for males and at the cervix for females, feel the sensation and chant *mooladhar* for a while. Move to swadhishthan in the cocyx at the base of the spine, feel it pulsate and chant *swadhishthan* for a while. Next, move to the manipur in the spine directly behind the navel — locate, feel and chant *manipur* for a while. Move to the anahat in the spine, directly behind the centre of the chest — locate, feel and chant *anahat*. Now come to vishuddhi in the spine directly behind the throat pit — locate, feel and chant *vishuddhi* for a while. Move to ajna at the very top of the spine, at the centre of the line directly behind the eyebrow centre. Locate and feel it pulsate and chant *ajna* for a while. Now locate the bindu where the Hindus keep a tuft of hair, feel the pulse and chant *bindu* for while. Finally come to the crown of the head and chant *sahasrar* for a while.

Now reverse the process, stopping, feeling and chanting at each one of the chakra. Practise five to ten rounds like this, increasing the speed a little every time. When you feel it is enough you can slowly come out of the process.

The process is very useful in developing awareness for all the chakras and laying a solid foundation for the arousal of the Kundalini. Practitioners can perform it under the instruction of a guru either directly or through a tape.

Preparation for Higher Practices

There is no method which is more powerful than kriya yoga exercises for evolving the consciousness. It is said to have been originally taught by Lord Shiv to his wife Parvati and has been communicated from teacher to practitioner only verbally so far. Modern age has brought these writings on paper now. It is important that one should have gone through hatha yoga exercises for about two years. The practitioner should have a thorough knowledge of the chakras and nadis and should have developed physical and mental awareness of them before starting the advanced exercises of kriya yoga. If this is not already done then the higher methods may be difficult to master and only little benefits may be drawn from their practises.

The best time for exercises is the divine period called *brahm-muhurt* exactly two hours before the dawn. This may vary from season to season and from country to country. Once it is located it can then be fixed for future. It is the time when food is digested properly and when one is not hungry, both the conditions being necessary for yoga. More importantly, spiritual and psychic forces are awake at this period and they are freely available as natural and unconscious vigour. One can try for oneself and see that the same practices at another time will be difficult to perform on one hand and little benefits will be drawn on the other.

Although there is a large number of kriya yoga exercises, nearing 80, only a selected set of them is presented here which is sufficient to evolve the consciousness to the required level or in other words, to raise the Kundalini. Each exercise should be learnt and developed one at a time every week, so that every week one more is added to the previous set. When the full set is developed, it may take between two to three hours to perform it.

However, everyone may not like all the exercises for one reason or the other and invariably a personal selection will prevail for each individual. Moreover, some may be able to devote the required time to each exercise, while some may be able to give only half time to each practice, depending on several factors. Taking all these things into account, an average time of two hours will be ideally required and sufficient for one's development. Thus the *brahm-muhurt* of two hours, for example, from 4 to 6 in the morning in many parts of India, is the ideal time. Similar timings can be found and fixed in different countries, as well as in different seasons in the same country.

One should avoid over straining oneself, that is, perform each exercise till you sweat and experience pain same thing applies, to respiration, that is, hold your breath as long as it is comfortable. Also, you may find it comfortable to breathe a little at the end of retaining the breath, before you exhale.

Latent higher powers are harnessed through the awakening of Kundalini. However, there are three *nadis*: Ida, Pingla and Sushumna. If Kundalini enters Ida, one may become overweight, develop emotional instability and psychic abilities, which may produce obstacles on the way to real spiritual progress. These are the signs of developing *kaph* and *ojas* in ayurveda. If the energy enters Pingla, one may experience excessive heat resulting in pride and a dominating attitude, which is also detrimental. These are the signs of developing *pitta* and *tejas* in ayurveda.

If the Kundalini fluctuates between the two nadis, it may result in fear, anxiety, insomnia, hallucinations, etc. These are the signs of developing *vatta* in ayurveda. Accordingly, the practitioner should notice carefully if any such signs are trying to develop in him/her, and then take corrective measures with the assistance of the guru or teacher.

Fresh and preferably vegetarian diet is recommended during the practise. Leftover food eaten for the second or third time gets devitalized which can block the subtle nerves and produce agitation. This will hamper the spiritual progress.

Alternatives to *brahm-muhurt* period of the morning, are an hour from half-an-hour before midday to half-an-hour after midday, and an hour before dusk. Drinking water and passing urine at the same time in continuation, or in the reverse order, should be avoided. This will avoid some urinary problems and make the urinary passages strong.

Advanced Kriya Yoga Exercises

Exercise 1 : Chakra Meditation
Sitting in siddhasana or siddha-yoni-asana, close the eyes and breathe normally. Beginning with mooladhar, move your awareness along the frontal passage of *arohan* to the frontal point of swadhishthan at the pubic bone, to manipur at the navel, to anahat at the centre of the chest, to vishuddhi at the throat pit, and to bindu at the point of the tuft of hair. Combine the movement of

awareness with the chanting of the mantras — mooladhar, swadhishthan, manipur, anahat, vishuddhi, bindu, for a couple of times at every chakra.

Now, reverse the process of shifting the awareness through frontal movement of *awarohan* from the bindu to mooladhar repeating the mantras mentally — ajna, vishuddhi, anahat, manipur, swadhishthan, mooladhar — as the attention halts at each centre. Having reached mooladhar at the end of the first round, start immediately on the second round of arohan beginning with swadhishthan and chanting the name of each chakra as you pass through it. On reaching the bindu, return through awarohan back to mooladhar immediately.

Continue with the rotation of awareness through ten rounds. The rotation should be rapid but without tension of locating the chakra, and without missing any of the centres. It should be as if you are glancing at the electric poles through the window of a fast moving train. One can facilitate the movement of awareness by associating it with a thin and sharp silver serpent moving along the path.

Exercise 2 : Nad Sanchalan or Sound Conduction

Sit in siddhasana or siddha-yoni-asana with eyes open. Exhale and bend the head forward making it drop down in a relaxed way. Take care that the chin is not pressing hard against the body. Bring awareness to the mooladhar chakra with a mental chanting of the word mooladhar. While inhaling, shift the awareness through frontal passage of *arohan*, to swadhishthan then, to

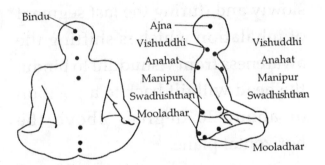

Bindu

Ajna
Vishuddhi
Anahat
Manipur
Swadhishthan
Mooladhar

Vishuddhi
Anahat
Manipur
Swadhishthan

Mooladhar

Nad sanchalan

manipur. Shift it from anahat to vishuddhi and then to bindu, chanting the corresponding names of the chakras as you pass through them. As you inhale, raise the head slowly and during the last segment of inhalation which is shifting the awareness from vishuddhi to bindu, the head will tilt back to a position of about 20 degrees above the horizontal plane.

Storing the breath inside and keeping the awareness at bindu level, keep chanting the mantra bindu, mentally. With the chanting of bindu, the power of awareness will build up and will suddenly explode into the vocal chanting of *Om*. This sound will carry you down to mooladhar through awarohan, the sound of O will be sudden, but the sound of M will be long drawn out, culminating like a buzz on arrival at mooladhar. The eyes which were fully open at bindu, will slowly close during the descent through awarohan, forming the *unmani mudra*. During descent the awareness of ajna, vishuddhi, anahat, manipur, swadhishthan, and mooladhar, should be maintained. On arrival at the mooladhar one should drop the head forward and open the eyes.

Chanting the word mooladhar, hold the breath, start the process of inhalation and ascension through *arohan* again. Chant the names of the chakras as you pass through them. Return to the mooladhar through *awarohan* as before. Complete 15 rounds in this manner, ending it finally at mooladhar.

Exercise 3 : Vayu Sanchalan or Breath Conduction
Sit in siddhasana with eyes closed and apply khechari mudra. Exhale completely and then bend the head

forward in an easy manner as before. Shift your awareness to mooladhar and chant mooladhar for a couple of times. While inhaling, begin the ascent through frontal passage of arohan, chant the word *arohan* mentally, and using the subtle *ujjayi inhalation*. Keep your awareness and chant the names of the chakras mentally as you pass through them, till you arrive at bindu with a tilted head. Keep chanting the mantra bindu.

Begin the return journey through awarohan, with *ujjayi exhalation*, and keep chanting the names of the chakras as you pass through them. During the descent, the eyes will close gradually, with a feeling of drowsiness, terminating into the *unmani mudra.*

Open the eyes, bend the head forward, and chant the mooladhar mentally a couple of times, and begin the ascent with subtle ujjayi inhalation for the second round. Complete 50 rounds with the ending at mooladhar keeping your eyes open. Remember that khechari mudra is to be maintained throughout this exercise.

Exercise 4 : Shabd Sanchalan or Word Conduction

Sit in siddhasana or siddha-yoni-asana with eyes open and use the khechari mudra throughout the exercise. Exhale and bend the head forward and concentrate on the mooladhar chakra for a while. Ascend the frontal passage of *arohan* with *ujjayi inhalation* and become aware of the sound of *so* which it makes. Be aware of the area associated with each chakra as you pass through till you arrive at bindu with a tilted head. Hold the breath for a while and concentrate on the bindu.

During the descent through the awarohan, be aware of the sound *ham* together with the area of each chakra as you pass through it, till you reach the mooladhar with *unmani mudra*. Open your eyes and lower your head. Repeat the process and complete 50 rounds.

Exercise 5 : Vipareet Karni Mudra or Flow Reversal
Adopt the Vipareet Karni Asana position which is similar to sarvangasana with the only difference that the body is held at an angle of about 45 degrees. Ensure that the chin does not press against

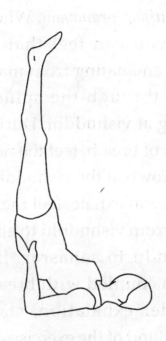

Vipareet karni mudra

the body and the legs are in a vertical position. Close the eyes and start the *ujjayi pranayam*. When you inhale, you can feel that warm nectar is emanating from manipur, flowing through the spine, and collecting at vishuddhi. During the retention of breath, feel the nectar is cooling down at the vishuddhi.

When you exhale, feel the nectar flowing from vishuddhi to ajna and from bindu to sahasrar, like an injection coupled with breathing. Soon after exhalation, start the second round of the exercise. Repeat the whole process and complete 20 rounds of it.

Exercise 6 : Advanced technique

Sit in siddhasana or siddha-yoni-asana with eyes open, make sure that one of the heels is pressed firmly in the direction of mooladhar chakra. Now apply the khechari mudra. Exhale and bend the head forward and chant mooladhar for a while. Ascend the frontal passage of *arohan* with *ujjayi inhalation*, remembering each areas as you pass through it, till you reach bindu through vishuddhi. Keep on chanting bindu mentally. Retain the breath inside, apply the moolbandh and shambhavi mudra. Repeat

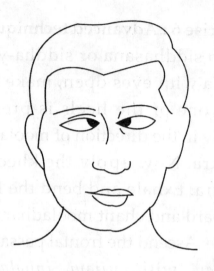

Shambhavi Mudra

s h a m b h a v i - k h e c h a r i - m o o l
mentally, while your awareness
passes through eyebrow centre; top
of the palate and mooladhar chakra,
respectively, as many times as you

can while holding the breath. Release the shambhavi mudra, and then the moolbandh. Now start the *ujjayi exhalation* from the bindu which should include the remembrance of each area till you reach unmani mudra at mooladhar. Bend the head forward and chant mooladhar. Start again with arohan and ujjayi inhalation and complete ten rounds.

Exercise 7 : Advanced technique
Sit in siddhasana or siddha-yoni-asana with eyes open, apply khechari mudra. Exhale and chant mooladhar for a while. Ascend

frontal passage with ujjayi inhalation till you reach the bindu while keeping your head tilted. Chant bindu and return with ujjayi exhalation to mooladhar in unmani mudra. Hold your breath while, applying tribandh (jalandhar, uddiyan and moolbandh) and nasikagra mudra. Chant the names nasikagra-uddiyan-mool with simultaneous attention at the three related points of concentration, as many times as is comfortably possible. Release the nasikagra mudra and tribandh, keeping the head down. With attention at mooladhar, chant mooladhar a couple of times. Repeat the whole process ten times.

Exercise 8 : Bindu Bhedan or Bindu Piercing

Sit in siddhasana/siddha-yoni-asana with your eyes closed, apply khechari mudra with head bent down and chant mooladhar. Ascend the frontal passage with ujjayi inhalation till you arrive at the bindu while keeping your head tilted. Apply the *yoni mudra* (closing ears with thumbs, eyes with forefingers, nostril with middle fingers, upper lip with ring fingers and lower lip with small fingers, in a gentle way). Apply moolbandh and vajroli mudra. Having thus closed the nine doors, concentrate on the spinal column and the bindu.

Visualize a copper trident or *trishul* — with the root in mooladhar, stem in the spinal column, and three sharp prongs rising up from vishuddhi. Feel that the trident is rising up and piercing the bindu over and over again. With each thrust, chant bindu-bhedan. Release the moolbandh and vajroli mudra, and open the nine doors. Putting the hands back on the knees, exhale the ujjayi way to mooladhar in unmani mudra and chant mooladhar. Complete five rounds of this exercise.

Care should be taken that the spine is straight and the vajroli mudra is applied properly in order to perceive the piercing sensation of bindu. A sort of electric shock can be experienced through the *vajra nadi* running to the brain.

Exercise 9 : Shakti Sanchalan or Conduction of Divine Force

Sit in siddhasana or siddha-yoni-asana with eyes closed, apply khechari mudra. Exhale fully and concentrate on mooladhar with bent head, and chant mooladhar. Ascend the frontal passage with ujjayi inhalation till you arrive at the bindu while keeping the head tilted. Retain your breath and apply yoni mudra, closing the nine doors. One can also apply moolbandh and vajroli mudra for slightly better results. Shift your awareness from bindu to ajna, from vishuddhi to anahat chakra at the spine, from manipur chakra at the spine, to swadhishthan chakra, and from mooladhar chakra, to frontal area of swadhishthan, to navel, and then

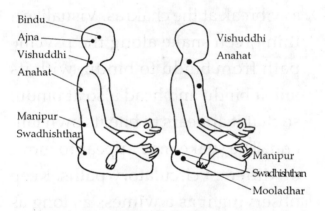

Shakti sanchalan

from there to the centre of the chest in the front to vishuddhi and to bindu thereby, completing the cycle in a continuous manner, without any break at the chakras. Visualize a thin green snake along the psychic path from bindu to bindu, with its tail at bindu and head also at bindu, so that it appears to bite its own tail-end. The snake may appear to move on different circulatory paths. Keep observing it as a witness as long as the breath can be retained. Then return to mooladhar in the usual *ujjayi* manner, ending in unmani mudra with a lowered head and chanting mooladhar. Complete five rounds.

Exercise 10 : Flowering the Sahasrar
Sit in siddhasana/siddha-yoni-asana with the eyes closed and apply the khechari mudra. Visualize a beautiful lotus flower with its roots at mooladhar, the stem extending through the spinal column, and the flower as a closed bud at the sahasrar. The colour of the roots and the petals at the bottom of the bud is light green. The main petals are pink and fine red veins are passing through them.

With your attention at mooladhar, exhale completely. Inhale with the help of ujjayi pranayam and carry your awareness from the roots through the stem to the bud. The journey should be similar to that of a caterpillar inside the stem, trying to reach the top. Retain your breath and keep the awareness inside the bud at sahasrar. You can also see the flower from outside. As you concentrate, it will begin to open and blossom into a full grown lotus with yellow pollen-tipped stamens and beautiful pink leaves.

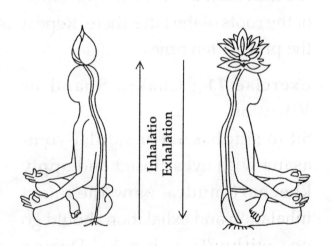

Inhalation
Exhalation

Flowering the Sahasrar

The flower may close and reopen a couple of times. At the end of retention of breath, descend down with *ujjayi exhalation* ending up at the mooladhar with the awareness of the roots of the lotus there. Repeat the process ten times.

Exercise 11 : Chakra Spand or Vibration

Sit in siddhasana or siddha-yoni-asana with eyes closed and apply khechari mudra. Now the ujjayi inhalation and exhalation should go on without a break. During exhalation, the awareness should be brought down to swadhishthan.

Inhale and carry the awareness to mooladhar first and then to the frontal passage of *arohan* till you reach the vishuddhi area. Start exhaling and carry attention from the vishuddhi area to the bindu, then to ajna and then on to swadhishthan. This is one round. One should aim at completing 20 such rounds, or more, depending on oneself.

Exercise 12 : Shaktipat or Infusion of Divine Energy
Sit in siddhasana or siddha-yoni-asana with eyes closed and breathe normally. Feel the presence of

divine hand on top of the crown centre. Visualize that "liquid white light with subtle energy" is emanating from the hand and is entering your body through the crown centre. Feel that every part of the head, the neck, the left shoulder, the left arm, the left hand and the right shoulder, the right arm and the right hand are filled completely to the end of the finger tips with this light. One can feel that both the hands seem to have become heavier and longer than before. One may experience hot or cold waves or vibrations, jerks, shocks or tickling sensations.

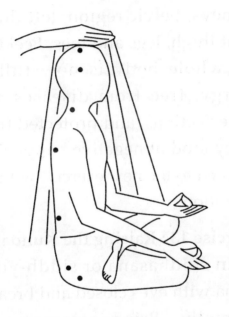

Shaktipat

Carry "liquid white light" to the lower parts through the spinal column, heart, lungs, spleen, liver, kidneys, pelvic region, left thigh, right thigh, legs and toes. Feel that the whole body is now full of energy, free from diseases and imperfections, and protected from every kind of negative happening. Proceed to the next exercise without repetition.

Exercise 13 : Raising the Kundalini
Sit in siddhasana or siddh-yoni-asana with eyes closed and breathe normally. Bring awareness to mooladhar chakra. Look at every

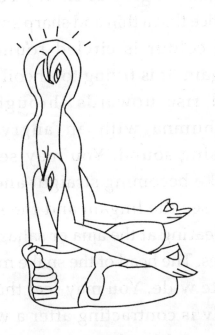

Raising the Kundalini

detail clearly and see the shiv-lingam in grey or smoky colour. Notice that a thin and sharp snake in red colour is circled round the lingam. It is trying to uncoil itself and rise upwards through the sushumna with an angry and hissing sound. You may see the snake becoming straight and one can see the lingam and the snake appearing at the ajna or sahasrar at times. The head of the snake may be quite wide. You may feel that the body is contracting after a while, followed by the ripples of bliss. Now there is no repetition, go to the next exercise immediately in continuation.

Exercise 14 : Witnessing the Astral Body

Bring awareness to the physical body, see that it is completely motionless and stiff like a stone. Become aware of the constant flow of natural breath. Stiffness of the body will go on increasing and along with it the awareness of breathing will also increase. The breathing may gradually become ujjayi, and khechari mudra may come into formation automatically. Become completely absorbed in

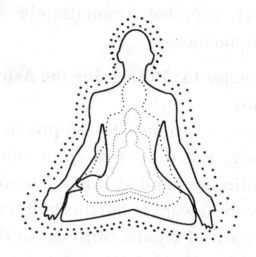

Witnessing Astral Body

breathing. You may notice that the body is expanding while inhaling and contracting while exhaling. What you see expanding and contracting is your astral body. With greater attention, the expansion and contraction will also become more sharp. The contraction of the body will finally reach the stage of reduction into a single point of light. Continue with the next exercise.

Exercise 15 : Witnessing the Self
Concentrate on the single point of light. The point will turn into a shining egg, and as you watch it, it will begin to grow in size and luminosity. Gradually the egg will take the shape of your body - the causal body - which is beyond the astral and physical bodies. It is pure Light - You are 'Self'.

Modern Research on Kriya Yoga Channels

Kriya Yoga is a very advanced technique of awakening Kundalini on the premise that there exists a system of channels or nadis or energy-flow in the whole body, which carries energy physically as well as mentally. The three main nadis—ida, pingla and sushumna are connected to thousands of small nerves which are spread throughout the human body for its nourishment and maintenance. These channels are not physical but causal and they can be known through their properties alone.

A vivid description of nadis has been given elsewhere, but the proof of their existence is to be attempted here, since their existence is the basis of the results of kriya yoga. Dr. Hiroshi Motoyama, a leading parapsychologist from Tokyo, has endeavoured in this direction. According to him, 'Asanas, mudras, pranayama and dharna are developed only through the knowledge of nadis. Acupuncture and concept of nadis have been running parallel to each other'.

Motoyama has found that the "triple heater system" in acupuncture and the five "pranas" of yoga represent the same thing. Lower heater below the navel, middle heater between the diaphragm and navel, and the upper heater between diaphragm and throat; in acupuncture correspond to apana, samana and prana, respectively, in yoga philosophy. "Governing vessel" and "conception vessel" in acupuncture correspond to the two "nadis" in yoga system. Several meridians in acupuncture start and

finish at the points where chakras
are located.

Proof of Existence

Dr. Motoyama has developed an "Apparatus for measuring the functional conditions of meridians and their corresponding Internal Organs," which proves the existence of nadis and chakras. The machine measures the currents in the body at a steady state and also under a shock from DC voltage. Fingernails and toenails are the acupuncture points where the charge is measured. These are the terminals for meridians from where the psychic energy enters and leaves the body: the points being called "Sei". He placed the electrodes on seven acupuncture points along the "triple heater meridian" along the back of the left arm and the front of the body, and at the right palm. On giving a 20 volt shock at the sei, on the tip of the fourth fingernail, the subject felt pain. After a few milliseconds, equal physical reaction was noted on all the electrodes, which was caused by the sympathetic nervous system in response to pain.

Motoyama then gave a painless and sensationless shock to the same point. After a few seconds, electrical responses were recorded at these specific points, which were connected to the "triple heater meridian": Palm electrode recorded no response while the greatest response was recorded at electrode on the other part of the meridian, just below the navel. This phenomenon has no explanation in physiology or neurology, but the claims made by acupuncture and yogic philosophy are validated. This proves the existence of nadis, since the movement of energy in the nadis and the meridian is much slower as compared with that in the nerves.

Dr. Nagahama of Chiba University Medical School observed that this happening clearly shows the existence of some other channel of transmission which is very well fitted by the description of the nadis.

Motoyama further proved that "prana" generates heat in the body. He coated the arm of a person with a special paint made of liquid crystals which would change colour with the change in temperature. Sei points, on stimulation for a few minutes by heat, changed colour along the meridian under stimulation.

It has been further noted that there is a kind of energy in the body which cannot be explained through neurophysiology. One can even record the physical counterpart of such an energy through experimentation. This shows that there exists a connection between the subtle and gross energies, although, one cannot exactly comment on the nature of the energy at present.

However, an important phenomenon is under observation which may show one day that there is a relation between energy and consciousness. This would tend to show that a yogi in whom generation of heat takes place as a result of "kriya yoga" and "kundalini yoga" practices, is also undergoing an upward revision of his/her consciousness.

Experiments of Motoyama measures three different states of nadi system:

- Baseline reading or steady state value of the body which exists all the time: This measure tells about the constitution in general.

- Body's reaction to mild and sensationless stimulation: This one tells about the reaction to events.
- After effects of stimulation : This one tells about the temporary functions of the body and resistances of the basic tissues.

A large number of experiments have been conducted in this direction. Most people are fond of existing in the normal range of values. Those with an abnormal range of values are found to be suffering from some disease. A couple of medical centres in Japan are using AMI machine of Dr. Motoyama for the detection of the diseases and their cures.

Yogis, too, are found to have abnormally high readings, but they do not suffer from any disease; it is the excess of "prana" or "ki" or "ch'i" which circulates in their nervous system as a result of yoga and meditative practices. This shows the reality of "psychic energy" which is found in the yogis. There is a complete balance between the ida and pingla nadis in the case of yogis, which is why they achieve freedom from diseases.

Ordinary people have an imbalance between the two nerves. If ida predominates, there is excessive cooling and therefore related diseases appear in the body.

Similarly, if pingla predominates, there is excessive heating and the related diseases show their presence in the body of the individual.

Balance is the key to good health and success. Balance between male and female principles is the prerequisite to Self-realization. This is what the ardha-naree-shwara (half Shiva, half Shakti) statue in the Indian temples convey. Same thing is told by the "hermaphrodite" gods in Greek mythology, and by the "androgynous" gods in early Christianity. Balance triggers God-realization, for which you learn Kriya Yoga.

Effects of Imbalance

Whereas the balance brings disease-free and healthy body, imbalance between ida and pingla is responsible for several diseases. The scientific/para-psychic research of Dr. Motoyama agrees with the yogic claim that the energy with physical and psychic properties flows within the human body.

According to the yogic philosophy there exists a direct relation between breathing and nadis. Breathing in the right nostril is related to pingla and the activities of the left hemisphere of the brain.

Similarly, breathing in the left nostril is related to ida and the activities of the right hemisphere of the brain. The flow of breath therefore, tells about the state of our body and mind. Pranayama is the art of breathing which brings the desired control and harmonizing conditions.

Considerable research has been done on the effects of breathing by Dr. I. N. Rige of Bucharest, Romania. He studied hundreds of patients and concluded:

- Those who breathed predominantly through the left nostril were prone to respiratory disorders, such as, chronic sinusitis; some loss in the sense of smelling, hearing and tasting; and could frequently suffer from pharyngitis, laryngitis, and tonsillitis; and chronic bronchitis.
- Left nostril breathers also suffered with intellectual weakening, gastroenteritis, headaches, poor liver and heart functioning, constipation, peptic ulcer, colitis, problems related to reproductive organs; for

example, irregularities of the ovaries and decreased libido.

- Those individuals in whom breathing predominated in the right nostril, were prone to hypertension. The situation was relieved on correction of the nasal deformities.

Dr. Motoyama's research also supports this conclusion. The whole research is in confirmation of the yogic philosophy, and the medical science can take a lot of clues about disease diagnosis from the philosophy of yoga. Swami Satyananda Saraswati (1984, 382) rightly observes that, "By controlling the speed, rate, rhythm, length and duration of the breath, by altering the ratio of inhalation to exhalation in the nostrils and by stopping the breath, we can activate or tone down neurological and mental processes so as to achieve heightened awareness and altered states of consciousness.

Constant practice of Kriya Yoga exercises given in the earlier sections, and pranayama in particular, brings the balance between the nadis and awakens the kundalini in due course of time.

One attains a disease-free body as long as he/she lives on earth, and it is a good-bye to further re-incarnations, if everything goes well.

About the Chakras

You are well conversant with the seven chakras or energy vortices in the body — mooladhar, swadhishthan, manipur, anahat, vishuddhi, ajna and sahasrar. Those living at the different levels of the chakras have different kinds of dispositions towards living the life.

- Someone living at mooladhar lives for a natural satisfaction of his/her instincts for greed, lust, anger, attachment and ego.

- One at the level of swadhishthan, lives for the satisfaction of desires, especially the ones related to sex.
- At the level of manipur one is concerned with the satisfaction of power instincts, though, of course, it is the boundary between the lower and the higher spiritual worlds.
- At manipur, one begins to turn towards philosophy of life, and eventually gets engaged in methods of spiritual evolution, in one way or the other.

- At anahat, one is tolerant, forgiving, compassionate, and has love for humanity in general.
- At the level of vishuddhi, one attains the power of speech, his/her body is rejuvenated through the awakening of the bindu, and he begins to knock at the door of liberation.
- At ajna, one's ego is fragmented into pieces, one experiences the death (of ego), resurrection opens the gate of liberation and one begins to receive direct commands from the inner guru.

However, individuals living at the level of lower chakras cannot understand those living at the level of higher chakras, since it is beyond their perception. It is just like the student at primary level of schooling who cannot comprehend mathematics or science or civics belonging to the level of graduation.

The situation is different for those at higher level of chakras. These are the individuals who have lived and transcended lower levels of instincts and have further awakened some higher centres of perception. They know how to act on demands of life and they understand and appreciate the mentality of persons living at lower levels of chakras.

Even at a particular chakra, there are different levels of evolution, just like finer divisions of a particular floor of a multi-storeyed building. For example, a person with freshly awakened *manipur* has love of power for self-gratification, while one with longer experience at *manipur* has learnt lessons and now uses power for constructive use of helping others rather than for destructive uses or for self gratification only. Each chakra is related to a particular gland, a set of nerves to serve and nourish the whole body. Relation of chakras with different parts of the brain and their functioning will now be discussed.

Findings of Neurosurgeons and Yogis

With the advances in technology on one hand and neuroscience on the other, it is now possible to study brain and the functioning of its various parts.

However, studying one's brain by one's own brain is like looking at one's eye through one's own eye, which may not be so simple and straight forward.

Nevertheless, scientists have studied brain objectively by

dissecting, photographing, X-raying, drugging for stimulation of circuits. On the other hand, yogis have carried out their study and research subjectively through yoga and meditation.

It is highly encouraging to know that the two different approaches have brought converging and agreeable results.

Thousands of years ago, when there was no science and modern microscopes, yogis described in exhaustive details the existence and functioning of seven chakras and three nadis and their offshoots. The so called science is now eventually confirming the findings of yogis. They do not yet have appropriate instruments and devices for the research on brain.

Yogis located chakras as points on the spinal column, where if attention is focussed and one meditates for considerable time, then some physical and phsychic experiences can be derived.

After a millennia of research, position of such points was fixed and confirmed. Now neuro-physiology and anatomy are slowly discovering glands and nerve plexuses which are connected to those points where chakras are supposed to exist. They are discovering that by controlling such positions one can control the metabolism of the body and hence the personality of the person.

Three Levels of the Brain

It is found that the brain of man is divided into three areas functionally, corresponding to three levels — reptilian, mammalian and human (MacLean, 1973). They are like three internally connected biological computers, each one having its own intelligence, subjectivity, memory and several other functions.

As the three names suggest, the three levels correspond to three evolutionary steps. They have different chemical compositions and different distributions of the neurochemicals in the brain. See figures 1 and 2. Findings of neuroscientists and yogis are very much in agreement with each other.

Reptilian Division

- This part takes care of our waking, conscious state.
- It controls mating, routine matters, obedience, slavish imitation, etc.
- It includes medulla oblongata and part of the reticular activating system.

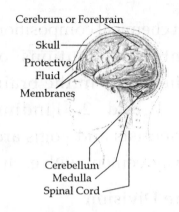

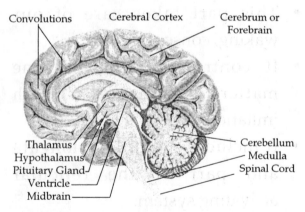

Section of the brain showing its inner parts
Figure 1

126

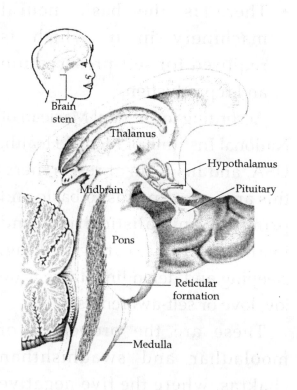

**Cross section of the brain stem
Figure 2**

- There is the basic neural machinery in it, which is required for self-preservation and reproduction.

According to Dr. Paul Maclean of National Institute of Mental Health, USA, and his team of researchers, this area corresponds to basic and primitive animalistic drives and instincts — living, eating, mating, sleeping and defending; there is no joy, love or self-awareness.

These are the properties of mooladhar and swadhishthan chakras, where the five negative sides are greed, lust, anger, attachment and ego. Dr. MacLean and his co-workers say that most of the people have their life dominated by this area.

This agrees very much with the yogic philosophy according to which most people live in mooladhar and swadhishthan chakras. Most of the life is spent in stimulating these two lowest chakras and satisfying the desires created by them.

Our daily functions are controlled by this primitive division which uses only 10 to 20 % of the brain, the rest of it containing higher centres remains asleep.

Yogis insist on stimulating these unused higher centres through yoga and meditation, so that the higher faculties of brain are awakened. This is where "kriya yoga" and "kundalini yoga" come into the picture.

According to psychologists there is a Mr. Hyde hidden beneath the sane facade of humans, which is containing things related to all that is animalistic and forbidden. Freud called it "id" from where arises the desires, passions and energy underlying our emotions and sense of existence.

According to psychologists there are two main centres in this area, located in the perineum and behind the pubic bone in the spine. These are exactly the locations of mooladhar and swadhishthan.

There is complete agreement between the psychologists and yogis on the point that most of the life is spent in stimulating these two centres and gratifying the desires created by them. Kriya yoga transcends this primitive area of lower centres of energy and awakens the higher centres.

Mammalian Division

- This is a level higher than the first, less ritualistic and more spontaneous.
- It controls emotion, memory and other behaviour.
- This is the subtler division on playful behaviour, awe and wonder.
- The structures here are under the control of the limbic system, which includes rage, fright, fear, revenge, anxiety, pain, joy, love and sex.
- These functions correspond to the activities of *manipur* and anahat chakras.

- On stimulation of the areas behind the navel and the centre of chest at the spinal cord, ripples are created and directed to the behavioral centres which are responsible for the related activities of the two chakras.

Human Division

- This is the highest of the three levels.
- It concerns the faculties of intelligence, thinking, analysis, discrimination, calculation, planning, intuition, creativity, speculation, scientificity, self

expression, artistic precision, cognition, etc.

- It is the newly evolved neocortex at work, represented by the frontal lobes of the brain.
- Some say that this itself is responsible for the highest class of perception, such as, knowledge, self awareness and higher consciousness.
- This is the force in the right direction with compassion for others and for the development of the society in the right way.
- A very important role which this division plays is in imparting the

knowledge of death and associated anxiety, which propels the person to live a better life on earth with spiritual goals in mind for perfection.

- It also helps in coping with the idea of dying.
- One who takes to yogic disciplines of kundalini yoga and kriya yoga, experiences death while still alive, in successful states of meditation, and the knowledge of beyond sets a goal to live and navigate in the remaining years in this incarnation.

According to David Loye (1982), frontal lobes are responsible for anticipation as well as looking into the future. The frontal lobes receive and pass information to both hemispheres of the brain, which in turn decide about what should be done and what not.

The research has confirmed the yogic view that those who can use both sides of the brain equally in a balanced way, get the best results physically as well as inwardly.

Thalamus and Ajna

According to physiology, there lies "Thalamus" at the top of the limbic system, in front of the pineal gland. Thalamus regulates the interaction of our senses and motor activity, which are caused by ida and pingla, in yogic terms.

Thalamus is also the main centre which regulates the pre-frontal cortex which includes the left and right hemispheres of the brain, which again are the domains of ida and pingla.

It also controls hypothalamus responsible for integrating and expressing emotions and regulating the endocrine glands. Cerebellum is also under the control of thalamus, which is helpful in controlling the movement.

To sum up, thalamus integrates thoughts, senses, emotions and action. It also recognizes pain, and is responsible for squeezing and contracting muscles and joints, in such situations.

Here is perhaps one of the most important points to be noted. Thousands of years ago, when there was no science at all, yogis declared the region between the eye-brows to be most important since the "ajna chakra" was situated just behind it. In yogic terms, ajna is the centre of command, compared to the biggest planet Jupiter, known as Brihaspati in Sanskrit.

Both functions of ida — sense and emotions, and both functions of pingla — motor and intellect, are found to meet here. In physiological terms the "high tension electric line" is charged here, and this has long been known as the central nadi — sushumna in yogic terms.

Ajna is the meeting point of ida, pingla and sushumna, which has physically been compared with the meeting point of the three rivers — Ganga, Jamuna and Saraswati at Prayag, the present day Allahabad in India.

It is the most important chakra, and yogis advice concentration on it with chanting of mantras so that once ajna is awakened, other chakras too are easily awakened. And whenever ajna is awakened, the gateway to liberation is opened. What more proof is required to show that science is following yogic discipline.

Centres in the brain have been defined by neurophysiology which correspond to the yogic description of chakras. Scientific description of thalamic area in front of the pineal gland corresponds to ajna chakra.

All these centres in the brain correspond to different layers of evolution within ajna. Hence awakening of a chakra on the spine, also awakens the corresponding centre in the brain, and the corresponding level of awakening in ajna is triggered too. Ajna therefore is the main commanding chakra.

Medulla oblongata corresponds to mooladhar area, and is directly connected with the pineal/thalamic area through nerves, which is the seat of ajna. Hence mooladhar and ajna are internally connected, which confirms the old yogic claim.

The awakening of one, triggers the awakening of the other automatically. However, if the lower chakras are awakened first, there are a couple of problems coming in. If ajna is awakened first, there are no serious problems and other chakras are easily awakened too.

As has been pointed out earlier, in most people only lower chakras are active and higher chakras are asleep. That is why people live and die ordinary animalistic life.

However, if ajna is awakened through yogic practices or otherwise, one lives a sort of philosophical or spiritual life, there is a purpose of living, and a desire to know the truth. Various techniques of awakening ajna have been given in the other book of this series *Chakras and Nadis*.

Kriya Yoga techniques, such as ajapa japa and others, create a psychic friction with the body which ignites the spark of higher consciousness.

It would be very much in place to give the example of boiling the water. It you lit a candle under vessel, it will never boil the water. Once a powerful heating device is used, water boils easily and converts into steam.

In the same way, when spiritual forces within the body are precipitated to the extent of boiling point, man is converted into god just as water is converted into steam. In the words of Swami Satyananda

Saraswati (1984, 398), "When the conditions for ignition reach the required temperature and pressure, energy is liberated within the body and mind, transforming our total personality."

Regarding the measurement of chakras, Dr. Hiroshi Motoyama has done pioneering work by developing certain machines. In his own words,

Fascinated... I too began physiological experiments about fifteen years ago to try to determine if chakras actually exist and to study their relationship to the autonomic nervous system and internal organs... Through various examinations we have been able to determine that there are significant differences in the physiological function of the organ associated with the chakra that the individual subjects claimed to have awakened. Therefore, this research has lead to the conclusion that chakras do, in fact, exist. (Motoyama, 1976, 6).

Concluding Remarks

The great sage Patanjali prescribed eight limbs of "raja yog": *yam, niyam, asan, pranayam, pratyahar, dharna, dhyan and samadhi.* The first four stages are covered by self-discipline and hatha yoga. As was said earlier, a period of two years of "hatha yog" would be ideal to prepare an individual for "kriya yog" practices. Kriya yog belongs to the next three stages, that is - *pratyahar* (withdrawal of senses from the world), *dharna*

147

(determination and concentration) and *dhyan* (meditation). Thus, kriya yog opens you to the last stage - *samadhi*, that is, absorption into the Absolute.

Dhyan (meditation) and *samadhi* (absorption) occur in an inseparable continuity. Just as one cannot say when childhood ends and youth begins, or when youth ends and old age begins, so, one cannot say when meditation ends and samadhi begins. It just happens in continuation. You only know about being in samadhi, when you come out of samadhi. And in samadhi too you pass from *savikalp samadhi* (absorption with fluctuations) to *nirvikalp samadhi* (absorption without fluctuations) in an inseparable continuity.

After devoting about two years on *hatha yoga* the practitioner should begin with *kriya yog* exercises. One week for each exercise, adding the other in the second week, would be the right way. You will keep asking questions until the kundalini is awakened; thereafter, you will begin to tread the unfrequented ways.

References

Motoyama, H. *A Psychophysiological Study of Yoga*, Institute for Religious Psychology, Tokyo, 1976, 6.

Motoyama, H. *The Mechanism Through which Paranormal Phenomenon Take Place*, Institute for Religion and Parapsychology, Tokyo, 1975, 2.

Motoyama, H. *Theories of the Chakras: Bridge to Higher Consciousness*, Quest, Illinois, 1981, 271-279.

Saraswati, Swami Satyananda,
Kundalini Tantra, Bihar School of
Yoga, Munger, Bihar, India, 1984.

OTHER TITLES IN THE SERIES